UNDERSTANDING YOUR
DIABETES

FOR PEOPLE WITH
INSULIN-
DEPENDENT
(TYPE 1) DIABETES

Acknowledgements

The author acknowledges with appreciation the constructive criticism of the many patients, nurses and other health professionals who helped to produce this book. Special thanks go to Eleanor Baldwin who provided nutritional information for this book.

UNDERSTANDING YOUR
DIABETES

DR PH WISE

MB, PhD, FRCP, FRACP
CONSULTANT PHYSICIAN IN ENDOCRINOLOGY

FOR PEOPLE WITH
INSULIN-
DEPENDENT
(TYPE 1) DIABETES

foulsham

LONDON • NEW YORK • TORONTO • SYDNEY

foulsham

The Publishing House, Bennetts Close,
Cippenham, Berkshire SL1 5AP, England

ISBN 0-572-02546-7

Printed in Great Britain by St. Edmundsbury Press, Bury St. Edmunds, Suffolk

Introduction

You may have had diabetes for some time; perhaps you already know much of what is in this book. On the other hand, the diagnosis may have just been made, and all that is involved in coming to terms with your condition may seem a little bewildering.

This book has been written to give you some idea of what diabetes is all about. It tries to answer the type of questions you will ask, both now and in the future, in order to help you understand and cope with insulin-dependent diabetes. It cannot cover the whole subject and makes no attempt to replace the advice and guidance of your physician. You will also find a list of further reading at the back of this book.

There is one thing that most authorities agree upon: the more that people with diabetes know and understand about diabetes, the better they will be able to control the condition and the healthier they are likely to be. Hopefully, this book will go some way towards achieving that, but never hesitate to ask for additional information and help whenever you feel you need it.

What is diabetes?

Diabetes is the name given to a disturbed chemical balance in the body, that can affect a number of different organs. About one person in every 50 is diabetic, although only about one out of every four people with diabetes actually needs insulin injections for treatment. The word diabetes comes from a Greek expression meaning 'siphon'. It refers to the increased urination and thirst that often occurs in newly diagnosed or uncontrolled cases. These symptoms are due to the high glucose content in the urine. This in turn results from an excessive build-up of glucose in the blood.

Diabetes is due to partial or complete lack of insulin. This hormone is normally released directly into the blood circulation from small pockets of cells called Islets of Langerhans, which are scattered throughout the pancreas gland (sweetbread). The pancreas rests in the upper abdomen, just beneath the liver, partly behind the stomach in the loop of the duodenum (see diagram opposite). The pancreas also produces enzymes, which pass through a duct into the duodenum, where they assist with the digestion of food. This part of the pancreas is only rarely affected in diabetes. Insulin in usable form was first extracted from animal pancreas in 1921 by two Canadians, Banting and Best. Shortly afterwards it proved successful in the treatment of human diabetes.

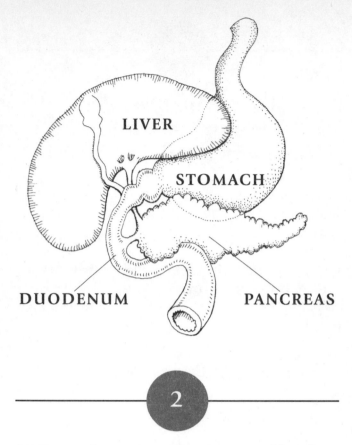

LIVER

STOMACH

DUODENUM PANCREAS

2

What does insulin actually do?

Insulin has many different effects, helping the body to manufacture proteins, fats and other substances. However, its main action is to encourage glucose in the blood to enter the cells of all major body tissues. In these tissues it can be stored in liver and muscle cells as a substance called glycogen. It can also be used to create energy and speed up chemical processes in the body.

If insufficient insulin is produced, the body accordingly malfunctions in a number of ways. Furthermore, since the glucose is not being used by the cells, it builds up in the blood to a level which is above normal. This is called *hyperglycaemia*.

What symptoms does uncontrolled diabetes (hyperglycaemia) produce?

When blood glucose rises above normal (see question 22 on page 35), a number of things may happen.

In the early stages, or if the rise of blood glucose is only moderate, there may be no symptoms at all. However, as the glucose level rises higher, one or more of the following may occur:

❖ The lens of the eye may alter its shape, producing **blurring of vision**.

❖ High glucose levels in the blood reduce the body's defences against infection. **Skin, urine, lung and other infections** may therefore occur. In fact, it may be just such an infection which first alerted your doctor that you might have diabetes.

❖ More glucose in the blood can interfere with brain activity, causing **poor concentration and lethargy**.

❖ By overflowing into the urine (where it is usually first tested), glucose may draw water with it; **more urine** is then passed.

❖ Excessive urination reduces the body's fluid reserves and stimulates **thirst** in an attempt to keep body fluid supplies normal.

❖ The passing of excessive urine also results in loss of essential chemicals (sodium, potassium and magnesium), producing **cramps, tiredness and weakness.**

❖ Because glucose cannot be properly used by the body and is lost in the urine, the body uses its stores of fat as a fuel supply, resulting in **weight loss.**

❖ If very severe loss of fluid occurs, the body becomes dry (dehydrated); **breathlessness and even coma** may then occur.

❖ Prolonged high levels of blood glucose, even if taking insulin, can damage body tissues over a period of years. This can lead to the so-called **complications of diabetes** (see question 29 on pages 46–9).

4

Why does diabetes develop?

There are different types of diabetes, but in many patients the tendency to diabetes is partly inherited from one or both sides of the family. However, there are almost always additional factors which are responsible for setting the disorder in motion.

In the more late-developing (non-insulin-dependent, type 2 or maturity-onset) diabetes, there may be only a mild deficiency of insulin. In such cases, diabetes may show up because of being overweight, or may result from the effects of repeated pregnancy, certain drugs, stress or just ageing itself. Diet alone or additional tablets are usually sufficient to control the blood glucose levels.

However, in cases such as yours, the lack of insulin is more severe or even total, perhaps resulting from additional severe damage to the pancreas gland by a virus, or from a variety of other factors. Therefore your diabetes is referred to as either insulin-requiring or insulin-dependent diabetes. Insulin is essential for treatment.

5

Does diabetes ever go away?

No. It can always be controlled and with treatment you should feel completely well. Even when treated, however, you must still carefully watch your condition and ensure that it is regularly reviewed by your doctor for the rest of your life.

6

What are the major aims and principles of diabetic treatment?

The first aim is to keep your blood glucose level as close as is practical to that of a non-diabetic person. By this and other means, the second aim can be achieved: to minimise or avoid the so-called complications of diabetes. There is a lot of research, from both Europe and the USA, which clearly shows that the more normal you keep your blood sugar, the less likely it is that you will develop these longer-term complications.

There are three essential principles for achieving good control: diet, insulin and exercise. The diet needs to provide a nutritious source of energy that is reasonably constant from day to day. The food you eat also needs to be accurately matched to a dose of insulin, which is usually injected twice or more daily. Exercise helps to keep body weight constant but in addition lowers the blood glucose level in a very similar way to insulin.

7

How is food normally processed by the body and what goes wrong in diabetes?

Foods – which are all different mixtures of carbohydrates, proteins, and fats – provide the body with energy. The energy value of any diet is expressed as calories:

❖ One gram of carbohydrate provides four calories.

❖ One gram of protein provides four calories.

❖ One gram of fat provides nine calories.

❖ One gram of pure alcohol provides seven calories.

Food also contains essential minerals and vitamins, but these do not provide the body with usable energy. Depending on age, weight and physical activity, the energy needs of the body range between 1,000 and 4,000 calories per day. After eating a meal, food passes into the stomach where it is digested (broken down) into smaller particles. Partly digested food then passes into the small intestine where digestion is completed and the small particles pass through the wall of the intestine into the blood stream.

The digested nutrients (carbohydrate, protein and fat) are carried to the liver where they may all be converted into glucose under some circumstances; however, most glucose comes direct from carbohydrate. Consequently, after a meal (especially if it is high in carbohydrate), there is a rise in the amount of glucose in the blood. The following diagram will give you an idea of the normal variation of blood glucose in a non-diabetic person. In people who do not have diabetes, a rise of blood glucose stimulates the pancreas to produce and release more insulin into the blood vessels which pass through the pancreas. From here, the insulin is distributed to the liver and all other body tissues.

Normal variation of blood glucose in a non-diabetic person

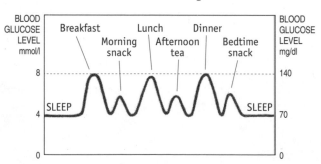

In this way, the glucose level is lowered back to normal within two hours, by forcing glucose to pass into body cells where it is processed to produce energy. If energy is not needed immediately, insulin allows glucose to be stored in muscles or liver in the form of glycogen (to be used later when extra energy may be needed), or promotes the production of fat (for more long-term storage). Insulin also stimulates the formation of proteins, important for the development of muscle, bone and other supporting tissues.

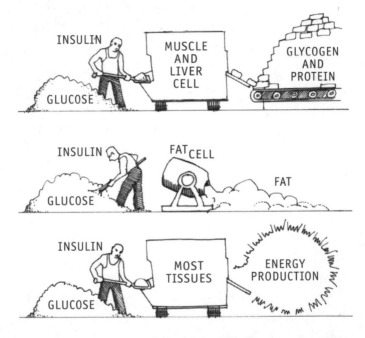

Because people with diabetes do not produce sufficient insulin, the blood glucose level is high even if no food is eaten. This is because the body makes glucose from its own stores of carbohydrates, proteins and fats. After a meal, the blood glucose level goes even higher. Some of this extra glucose is removed from the blood by escaping through the kidneys into the urine. Furthermore, since the body cannot use the glucose properly to produce energy, such energy must be obtained by other means: from the breakdown of fat stores and protein-rich tissues in the body. This process leads to the loss of weight and ill health of uncontrolled diabetes.

What are the principles of diabetic diets?

A diabetic diet is a healthy, balanced diet: the sort of diet that is recommended for everyone (although very young children and babies have special requirements). Why not convert your family and friends? Your dietitian, ideally also involving some members of your family, will tell you about foods which will suit both your likes and needs, whatever your ethnic or national background. There is no need to buy 'special' diabetic foods; they are more expensive, and not necessarily more healthy.

Some foods cause problems by causing a very large rise in blood glucose. They are then said to have a high glycaemic index (GI). In general there are alternatives that are healthier, not only for people with diabetes but for good nutrition generally. Your dietitian will explain this to you in more detail, and will be able to provide you with a list that will help you to choose foods of low glycaemic index. There are six general principles that all people with diabetes should follow to keep their diabetes well controlled.

Reduce sugar and sugary foods.

We are talking mainly about glucose itself, jam, honey, sweets, chocolates, fizzy (sugary) drinks and fruit squashes or juices. These foods cause a rapid rise in blood glucose which is difficult for insulin to deal with. Many foods contain sugar (chemical name: sucrose). We now know that sucrose has quite a low glycaemic index and only makes your blood glucose go half as high as glucose itself. However, sucrose gives you 'empty calories' – they have very little nutritional value. It is therefore wise to avoid foods in which sugar is the major ingredient. Check the ingredient label of a food if you are not sure whether it is suitable. The ingredients are listed in order of weight, so if sugar is at the top of the list it means the food contains a large amount. If sugar is towards the end of the list, the food is suitable as it will contain very little sugar. Artificial sweeteners are safe, but you should avoid those that are combined with sugar.

Eat regularly.

You should aim for three meals a day. One or two large meals raise the blood glucose too high and are difficult for insulin to deal with properly. A meal may be as little as a sandwich, or as much as a cooked meal of meat, potatoes and vegetables, followed by dessert. Eating regularly is particularly important to **avoid hypoglycaemia** (low blood sugar).

As you can see in the tables in question 11 (see page 22), different insulins have different times of peak action and duration. The type and dose of insulins you have been prescribed will have been chosen to suit your lifestyle and requirements. Check with your diabetes nurse, doctor or dietitian to find out whether your insulin regimen requires you to eat snacks between meals.

Eating a larger meal than usual is fine, on occasions, but you will need to increase your insulin dose before that meal to prevent the blood glucose from rising too high. Your diabetes nurse, doctor, or dietitian will be able to advise you on this.

Eat some starchy food with each meal.
In earlier years, people with diabetes were advised to avoid or restrict all starches. We now know that a certain intake of starches is important. They are broken down into sugar by the body. The healthier types are broken down more slowly than sugary foods, causing a slower, smaller rise in blood glucose. Some starches should be included in each meal. Boiled potatoes, oatmeal or multi-grain breads, oat-based cereals such as porridge, All Bran and muesli and brown rice are the ones to go for. Hypoglycaemia (see question 24 on page 38) may occur if you forget to include these foods or try to reduce them drastically.

However, you should note that white bread and baked potatoes have a very high glycaemic index; avoid them! These foods, together with white rice and some refined cereals like cornflakes, are likely to contribute to poor diabetic control. They may well cause weight gain as well.

Eat less fat and fatty foods.
We are including here butter, oil, margarine, all fried foods and pastry of all types. Having a high fat intake increases your risk of suffering from heart attacks or strokes, which are in any case rather more likely to occur in someone with diabetes. Smoking or being overweight

increases the risk still further. It makes sense to cut down risks! Cutting down on fat has the added advantage that it automatically reduces your calorie intake. Weight for weight, high-fat foods may have as many as twice the number of calories as non-fat or low-fat alternatives. Avoiding high-fat foods will therefore help you to reduce your weight, if necessary, or help to prevent you from becoming overweight.

Drink alcohol in moderation.

There is no uniform agreement on safe alcohol limits, however safe weekly limits are generally considered to be 15–18 units for a woman, or 22–28 units for a man, spread over the week. One unit is a single pub measure of spirit, an average glass of wine or a half pint of beer, lager or cider. Alcohol is high in calories and will make you gain weight. Too much of it is also bad for your liver, heart, brain and nerves. The actual amount of alcohol that will cause damage to different people will vary considerably, however.

Alcohol excess is particularly harmful if nerve damage from diabetes is already present (see page 47). Too much alcohol at once, especially on an empty stomach, may actually cause your blood glucose level to go too low. **Do not drink alcohol on an empty stomach**, avoid having more than three or four drinks in a session, and follow alcohol with a snack containing at least some starchy food, such as a sandwich. This is very important at bedtime to avoid low blood glucose levels overnight.

Eat more fibre.

Dietary fibre is the part of a plant that is not digested properly by the body. High-fibre foods include multi-grain bread, brown long-grain rice (which has a lower glycaemic index than white rice), wholegrain pasta, vegetables (especially beans, peas, and lentils) and wholegrain breakfast cereals. Eating high-fibre foods with your meals reduces the rise in blood sugar that occurs after eating. High-fibre foods can also be helpful in reducing blood cholesterol, and also tend to be quite filling. They can therefore be helpful in reducing weight and preventing weight gain. They also help to produce regular bowel movements.

Not being overweight has already been mentioned several times in this section. The table on page 19 shows the desirable weight for different heights. It is very important that you try to reduce your weight if you are overweight. Diabetes is more difficult to control when you are overweight. If you are having difficulty in losing weight, ask your doctor to refer you to the dietitian, who will draw up a personal eating plan to help you to achieve your weight target.

It is very important to see a dietitian regularly; you will be given too much information to remember at your first visit. Furthermore, your diet may need to be changed over a period of time, particularly if you change your way of life, gain weight, or if the type of insulin you use is changed. Use page 59 to note your dietitian's contact number.

9

Is weight control important?

Yes, very much so. Being overweight increases your need for insulin and can make your diabetes less stable. It also raises your cholesterol and other fat levels. It may cause or aggravate conditions unrelated to diabetes, such as high blood pressure and arthritis. The only way you can influence your weight is by diet and exercise (see question 14 on page 27). Remember that one extra hour of brisk walking (or half an hour of continuous swimming, jogging or squash) each day will almost predictably allow you to lose about 7 kg (15 lb) in a year – providing you do not increase your food intake! Use the table below as a guide to your goal weight.

Guide to healthy weight range for adult men and women

HEIGHT		HEALTHY WEIGHT RANGE	
4' 10"	146 cm	6 st 10 lb–8 st 4 lb	43–53 kg
4' 11"	149 cm	7 st 0 lb–8 st 8 lb	44–55 kg
5' 0"	152 cm	7 st 4 lb–9 st 2 lb	46–58 kg
5' 1"	154 cm	7 st 7 lb–9 st 5 lb	47–60 kg
5' 2"	157 cm	7 st 10 lb–9 st 12 lb	49–63 kg
5' 3"	160 cm	7 st 13 lb–10 st 2 lb	50–64 kg
5' 4"	162 cm	8 st 4 lb–10 st 7 lb	52–67 kg
5' 5"	164 cm	8 st 7 lb–10 st 10 lb	53–68 kg
5' 6"	166 cm	8 st 10 lb–11 st 0 lb	55–70 kg
5' 7"	169 cm	8 st 12 lb–11 st 5 lb	56–72 kg
5' 8"	172 cm	9 st 0 lb–11 st 10 lb	58–75 kg
5' 9"	175 cm	9 st 4 lb–12 st 0 lb	59–77 kg
5' 10"	177 cm	9 st 8 lb–12 st 6 lb	61–79 kg
5' 11"	179 cm	9 st 12 lb–12 st 8 lb	64–80 kg
6' 0"	182 cm	10 st 2 lb–12 st 12 lb	65–82 kg
6' 1"	184 cm	10 st 7 lb–13 st 4 lb	67–84 kg
6' 2"	187 cm	10 st 12 lb–13 st 10 lb	69–87 kg

Figures given are for a recommended body mass index (BMI) of 20–25 calculated as weight (in kg) divided by height (in metres)^2.

How is insulin given?

Insulin needs to be injected because if it is taken by mouth the digestive enzymes of the stomach and intestine destroy it before it can be absorbed. The amount of insulin used in treatment is expressed in units. Insulin is manufactured in various strengths (concentrations) throughout the world, but these days 100 units per ml is the one most often used. It is important to check your insulin each time it is prescribed and dispensed to make sure that you have the correct type. It should always be kept cool (but never frozen), preferably in a domestic refrigerator.

What are the differences between the various types of insulin?

Soluble, clear or regular insulin (including lispro insulin) consists of the pure hormone the action of which has not been prolonged by any additive. Insulin used to be extracted only from beef pancreas. Nowadays, the main insulins used are of pork origin, or more commonly synthesised artificially to resemble human insulin exactly. The length of action depends on the dose given but is rarely longer than 8–10 hours, so that three injections of this type of insulin would need to be given each day to control the blood glucose level adequately. The higher the dose, the greater the lowering effect on blood glucose. The same applies to all the other types of insulin described later. With the exception of lispro insulin (Humalog), higher doses also mean a more prolonged effect.

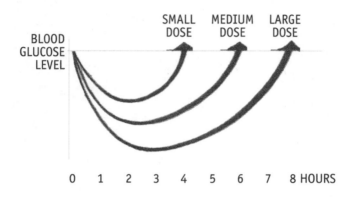

Insulin can be linked to various proteins which prolong its action to between 12 and 36 hours, depending on the type and dose used. By contrast with soluble insulin, these **longer-acting insulins** are usually cloudy and mostly need to be given only once or twice a day. Some insulins are biphasic (mixture of short and long-acting insulins) and often provide better control.

Although different manufacturers produce very similar insulins, once control has been achieved, it is wise to keep to the same manufacturer since minor changes may alter your reaction. Always check the insulin carefully as soon as it has been dispensed by your pharmacy, since errors can occur.

Short-acting insulins

Insulin name	Origin	Onset (mins)	Peak (hours)	Duration (hours)
Actrapid	Human	20–30	3–4	6–10
Hypurin neutral	Beef or pork	20–30	3–4	6–10
Velosulin	Pork	20–30	2–3	6–10
Humulin-S	Human	20–30	2–3	6–10
Humalog	Human	5	1–2	5–6

Intermediate-acting insulins

Insulin name	Origin	Onset	Peak (hours)	Duration (hours)
Humulin M1-M5	Human	20–30 mins	2–8	20–24
Mixtard 10, 20, 30, 40, 50	Human or pork	20–30 mins	4–6	20–24
Insulatard	Human or pork	1–2 hours	5–8	20–24
Humulin-I	Human	1–2 hours	6–8	18–24
Hypurin Isophane	Beef or pork	1–2 hours	6–8	18–22
Humulin Lente	Human	20–30 mins	8–12	22–30
Hypurin Lente	Beef	20–30 mins	8–10	22–30
Lentard MC	Beef or pork	20–30 mins	8–12	22–26
Human Monotard	Human	20–30 mins	8–11	20–24
Hypurin Biphasic	Pork	30 mins	4–12	20–24

Long-acting insulins

Insulin name	Origin	Onset (hours)	Peak (hours)	Duration (hours)
Humulin ZN	Human	2–4	10–14	24–30
Hypurin Protamine Zinc	Beef	2–4	14–16	28–34
Ultratard	Human	2–4	10–18	28–34

At *what times should insulin be given?*

Insulin should always be injected 15–30 minutes before meals. The only exception is lispro insulin (Humalog). Its action begins within five minutes, so that it can (and should) be given immediately before a meal. It can also be given during or even on completing a meal. This is useful if you are not sure how much food you will be eating! Giving an injection too early may result in blood glucose levels falling too low before food is absorbed into the bloodstream; this is particularly important when short-acting insulins are being used. Injecting too close to the start of a meal with any insulin other than lispro (Humalog) may result in blood glucose rising too high before the insulin has a chance to act. Both situations are clearly undesirable.

Once-daily injections are rarely able to control the blood glucose level for a whole 24 hours. However, some people with type 2 diabetes who need insulin as well as blood glucose-lowering tablets may be offered a single daily dose of medium-acting insulin at bedtime. This ensures that they start the day with more normal blood glucose levels.

Twice-daily injections (before breakfast and evening meal) often work well. A somewhat higher dose is usually needed for the morning injection. Mid-morning, mid-afternoon and bedtime snacks are needed to 'buffer' the action of insulin in both once-daily and twice-daily routines.

Three short-acting doses each day before meals, together with a medium- or long- acting insulin at bedtime (and sometimes in the morning as well) has the advantage that the doses can be changed from day to day to allow for different meal sizes and patterns of exercise. Timing of meals and exercise can also be much more flexible. Mid-morning and mid-afternoon snacks can usually be omitted – although the **bedtime snack is still essential.** Many people find that on this regimen, dose adjustments are easier to plan and more logical.

13

How are the injections of insulin given?

The only syringes now in use are plastic disposable ones, with fixed needles now almost standard. Many doctors feel that a disposable syringe and needle can be re-used quite safely, but check that your doctor agrees with this approach. If so, after injection, replace the syringe in its plastic envelope without rinsing it and keep it in the refrigerator. After five or six injections, a new syringe and needle should be used, although blunting of the needle may mean changing it more frequently. Syringes vary both in capacity (30, 50 or 100 units) and in markings, which can be confusing. You should always confirm with your doctor or nurse exactly how the marks on the syringe correspond to the dose to be injected.

Drawing up insulin

Draw back the same amount of air into the syringe as the quantity of insulin you will need to draw up. Inject air into the ampoule. Slowly, draw back the quantity of insulin required. If an air space or bubbles develop, move the plunger in and out until the correct amount of insulin, free of bubbles, is in the syringe. Then withdraw the needle. Different types of short- and long-acting insulins are sometimes prescribed to be given at the same time. Draw up the clear insulin first, then the cloudy, and inject as soon as possible.

Insulin pens

Many people now prefer the convenience of pens which can be 'loaded' with a cartridge containing 150 or 300 units of insulin. Pens are also available preloaded with insulin; once empty, you simply discard the pen and start a new one. With all pens, the dose is 'dialled-up' before injection, making for a simpler injection routine. The special needles are detachable, so that they can be changed as often as necessary. Most insulin types are now available in cartridge form. It is always a good idea to have a spare pen in reserve in case the ones you are using are broken or mislaid.

Injection technique

This is always best demonstrated by the doctor or nurse. Cleaning the skin with spirit before injecting is no longer thought to be necessary. Spirit tends to toughen the skin, making injections more difficult and blunting your needles more quickly. Injections should be given under the skin, not into it, using a needle no longer than 12 mm (½ in). Shorter needles of 8 mm (⅜ in) or 5 mm (¼ in) are also available and may suit you better. The injection should ideally be given at right angles (90°) to the skin surface, but certainly at no smaller angle than 45°. The needle can be inserted to the hilt. Never use exactly the same spot twice in succession, although different spots no closer than 2–3 cm (1 in) apart in the same area can be used successfully. Ideally, rotate the injection sites so that a different major area of the body is used for each injection. Repeated injecting in the same area is more likely to produce swelling (hypertrophy) or occasionally loss (atrophy) of fat tissues at the site of the injection. However, the purity of the insulins which are now used makes this problem far less likely to occur. All diabetic people develop their personal routine, but the diagram below shows the range of possibilities.

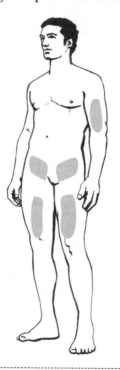

In some people, insulin seems to have a more rapid effect if injected into the arms than the legs, and with a faster but more steady effect if injected into the wall of the abdomen. Your own experience may lead to the use of certain areas rather than others.

Some stinging during the injections is usual. Pain or burning after the injection and irritation or reddening at the site of the injection are abnormal, and should lead to discussion with your doctor. The cause may be either faulty injection technique or an allergy to the type of insulin being used.

When going to your doctor or the pharmacy, always take both a syringe (or your injection pen) plus an empty insulin package or ampoule along, to compare this with what is being newly prescribed or supplied. This will help to avoid errors.

14

Is exercise important?

Yes. Any form of exercise causes the muscles to use more glucose. Blood glucose level is lower immediately after exercise. There is also a longer-term lowering, with less swings, in the levels of blood glucose in people whose lifestyle is more energetic. Taking exercise often means that you need to reduce your insulin dose beforehand, or increase your intake of food. In some people, the blood-sugar lowering effect of insulin continues for many hours after the exercise. It may then be necessary to reduce the next dose of insulin to allow for this effect. Only trial and error will allow you to work out what is best for you. Most people do not realise how inactive they really are. Tiredness and fatigue after a day's work are more likely to be due to emotional stress and tension than to the effects of muscular exercise.

Any type of exercise is good for people with diabetes, including cycling, regular sport or just walking. A careful look at your lifestyle and discussion with friends and family should help you plan a more energetic way of life, whatever your age or condition. Remember that many factors can affect the blood glucose level. This diagram will remind you of the most important ones.

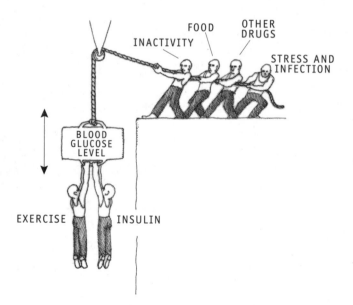

Can exercise cause any problems?

Yes. If both food intake and insulin dose remain the same, a sudden increase in exercise can result in quite a sudden fall of blood glucose, producing an insulin reaction (hypoglycaemia or 'hypo'). This is because exercising muscle uses up some of the glucose in the blood. In addition, if you exercise the legs (by cycling, for example) after an injection into a leg, the insulin is absorbed into the circulation more quickly. This can lower the glucose level in the blood even further. The symptoms will be described later in this book (see question 24 on page 38).

When exercising, hypos can be prevented by:

❖ Eating a larger meal (or a portion of starchy food) before exercise, or nibbling during exercise.

❖ Reducing the insulin dose immediately preceding the planned exercise (for example, with a game of squash) by an amount which your doctor will advise, or you will work out yourself by trial and error.

❖ Always carrying a small carton of fruit juice, lumps or cubes of sugar, or a glucose tablet such as Dextrosol in case a hypo occurs, or to prevent one should the exercise prove longer and more strenuous than anticipated.

What is the 'honeymoon' phase of diabetes?

In some people with diabetes, the insulin dose falls during the first few weeks or months of treatment. Occasionally insulin can be stopped altogether. However, this is only temporary and does not indicate that your diabetes is cured. Watch your blood tests carefully and be prepared to recommence the insulin. Why some people experience this event is still not clear.

Why is it necessary to control diabetes well?

It is not hard to put together a pattern of diet, insulin, and exercise in such a way as to avoid the symptoms of both hyperglycaemia (see question 3 on page 8) and hypoglycaemia (see question 24 on page 38) – but this is not enough! Particularly if you are young, with a long life span ahead, keeping blood glucose levels as close as possible to those of a non-diabetic has now been shown by many research workers to reduce the likelihood of getting the so-called complications of diabetes in later life. These are dealt with later (see question 29 on pages 46–9). Achieving good control requires a lot of your own involvement and thought, and your doctor or diabetes nurse will be glad to provide additional guidelines on the many small ways for improving control.

How can I tell whether my diabetes is well controlled?

Certainly not by the way you feel! Many people with diabetes may feel perfectly well, despite having uncontrolled diabetes. However, you should be able to recognise easily the symptoms listed in question 3 (page 8). If any of them occur, your diabetes is seriously out of control. The cause must be found and corrected immediately.

By testing the urine?
This is not really ideal. The glucose content of urine does not accurately reflect the rapid changes in blood glucose that are found in people having insulin for their treatment. Testing urine is only second best.

By testing the blood?
Yes! Measuring your own blood glucose is now very simple and is so much more informative than testing urine. Only one drop of blood is needed. When placed on a special strip, a patch changes colour according to the glucose level. More accurate readings can be obtained by using pocket-size and inexpensive meters. These give a digital read-out, and many meters

have memory banks for keeping the results. Some even allow you to feed the results into a computer so that a print-out can be generated. These accurate techniques enable you to assess and control your own diabetes yourself to a degree which was previously impossible. Your doctor or nurse will be happy to discuss these procedures with you. Untreated or poorly controlled diabetes also raises the blood level of certain fats (lipids), including cholesterol and triglyceride. Your doctor will check the blood levels of these fats from time to time and may advise a change in diet and sometimes fat-lowering drugs, if they are abnormal. There is now considerable evidence to suggest that keeping blood fats at normal levels improves the long-term health of arteries (see page 46).

A blood test (called **haemoglobin A1c or HbA1c**) provides an estimate of what your average blood glucose has been over the previous two to three months. It is a very useful way of helping your doctor assess your overall glucose control. A person without diabetes usually has levels less than 6 per cent. In someone with diabetes, a haemoglobin A1 value above 7–7.5 per cent usually means that there is room for improvement. The fructosamine test is used by some doctors. It measures how well your diabetes has been controlled over a shorter period of 10 to 14 days.

How is blood tested for glucose?

A small drop of blood, sufficient to produce a proper 'blob' (not a smear) on the blood testing strip, is the first essential. Using a lancet in one of the readily available 'prickers' is the best way to get the blood painlessly and reliably. Use all the finger tips in turn to avoid soreness, and consider using the sides of fingers or the earlobes if fingertips do become sore! Whichever the type of strip used, the **exact** moment that the blood comes in contact with the strip must be accurately noted (or the button on the meter pressed). If blood has to be wiped off the strip again, **accurate timing is essential.** Some meters will time your test automatically from the moment the blood touches the strip. If you use a meter, you can also get 'check fluids' to see if your meter gets the right reading. Or ask your doctor or nurse to cross-check a blood sample in the laboratory from time to time to see if it matches your reading. If you use a meter to read the sticks and get an unusually high or low reading, check the colour visually (if it is that sort of strip); a meter can be faulty!

When should tests be done?

You should aim to do at least one test a day, testing at different times each day so that you and your diabetes advisers can get a proper picture of your control. Without this feedback you have no way of knowing if you are properly controlled. You will also not know whether any dose changes you are (or should be) making are having the desired result. It is impossible to overstate the importance of ensuring that your blood glucose levels are as close as possible to those of a non-diabetic person.

Why is it so important to keep my glucose levels normal?

All research now points to the fact that the lower the glucose levels, the greater the likelihood of remaining free of complications – and if they occur at all, the milder they will be. This applies to eye and kidney problems, as well as to nerve and artery damage. The large US Diabetes Control and Complications Trial (DCCT) has confirmed other smaller research trials in proving that keeping your HbA1c below 7.5 per cent will make an enormous difference to your long-term health prospects, with less risks of retinal, kidney and nerve damage. Lower blood glucose levels do mean a slightly higher risk of hypos. However, if you follow the guidelines in this book, this should rarely be a major problem.

What is a normal blood glucose level?

In people without diabetes, fasting blood glucose (after not eating overnight) is less than 5 millimoles per litre, or 90 milligrams per decilitre (shortened to mmol/l or mg/dl). After food, it rarely rises above 8mmol/l (145mg/dl). In untreated or uncontrolled diabetes, blood glucose may even rise above 30mmol/l (540mg/dl). With treatment, your doctor will aim to keep your level at less than 10mmol/l (180mg/dl) for all or most of the time and will often help you to achieve lower levels: 4–7mmol/l (70–125mg/dl) before meals, and 7–10mmol/l (125–180mg/dl) one to two hours after meals. It is important to emphasise that symptoms of hyperglycaemia (question 3 on page 8) rarely occur unless blood glucose is consistently higher than 14mmol/l (250mg/dl).

It cannot be said often enough that just because you feel well, it does not necessarily indicate that your diabetes is controlled.

How can I achieve the best possible control of my diabetes?

This is probably one of the most important challenges facing a person with insulin-dependent diabetes. It is not easy because our lifestyle varies so much during a single day, and from one day to the next. A normal pancreas adjusts to diet, exercise and stress automatically by changing its output of insulin. Having diabetes, you have to take over this function.

Firstly, always have three regular meals each day. A mid-morning and mid-afternoon snack are usually necessary if you are on a twice-daily insulin regimen. A before-bedtime snack is essential whatever insulin regimen has been advised for you. It won't hurt to go out once in a while for a meal that might be larger than usual, but **anticipate** any problems by taking more insulin beforehand. Be prepared to do fingertip blood sugar tests after such an unusual meal: this will tell you whether you have adjusted your dose correctly. Remember that two hours after a meal blood glucose should not often exceed 10mmol/l (180mg/dl). The same anticipation applies to stressful situations and to infections of all types. Don't wait for diabetes to go out of control; raise the dose as soon as you anticipate a problem and check the blood glucose to see whether you have reacted to the situation correctly. Look again at the pulley diagram on page 28 to remind yourself of the factors which will affect your blood glucose level.

The same **anticipation** is the keynote to handling exercise (see also question 14 on page 27). Drop your insulin dose by anything from four units to half of your usual dose before a game of tennis or squash, a cycle ride or even a brisk hike. Taking some extra carbohydrate with exercise may, of course, suit you better. You may find that you need to do both. Always check your blood glucose level to see that you have done it correctly. Remember that on two doses of insulin each day, your morning dose affects the blood glucose at midday and before the evening meal, while your evening dose affects the late-night and early-morning glucose levels. On four doses of insulin a day, each pre-meal dose is reflected by the blood glucose level four to six hours later, and the bedtime dose affects the early-morning blood glucose level. If you can achieve before-meal blood glucose levels of 4–7mmol/l (70–125mg/dl) and after-meal levels of 7–10mmol/l (125–180mg/dl) for most of the time, you can be very proud of yourself.

Even if you get the most accurate blood glucose result, it will only improve your control if you act on it! Therefore, do your one or two tests a day, and record the results together with any unusual happenings (such as insulin reactions) in your test record book. Then be prepared to adjust, as outlined above, all the variables of your lifestyle and insulin doses. If you get an unusual result, ask yourself at the time why you think it happened, and again write the reason down in your record book. It will help you to understand your diabetes better. Contact your doctor or nurse as often as you think necessary. Do not wait until your next appointment before getting this advice, otherwise you will have lost valuable time.

What is hypoglycaemia, insulin reaction or hypo?

When the blood glucose level falls below 3mmol/l (55mg/dl), the following symptoms may develop:

❖ hunger

❖ dizziness

❖ sweating

❖ trembling

❖ palpitations

❖ slurring of speech

❖ faintness

❖ confusion and vagueness

❖ loss of consciousness and fits

A hypo occurring at night may reveal itself only by restlessness, nightmares and a headache the morning after. Sometimes you will find a surprisingly high blood glucose the morning after a hypo: a rebound sometimes known as the Somogyi effect or dawn phenomenon. A positive ketone (see question 26 on page 41) but negative glucose test in the first urine passed next morning is another clue to a hypo occurring during the previous night. Every diabetic has a slightly different pattern of symptoms of hypoglycaemia; in fact your doctor may deliberately arrange to give you a hypo to help you recognise the symptoms, should they occur later.

After many years of having diabetes, the early warning hypo symptoms – which consist of sweating, trembling and palpitations – may be lost. This problem may also result from having your diabetes too well controlled. If this happens, you will need to be more alert to the other symptoms or slacken off your control a bit. A slight reduction of insulin doses or change of insulin type may be worth a try, after discussing it with your doctor. This maneouvre may restore the usual warning symptoms.

The main causes of hypoglycaemia are as follows:

❖ **Late or missed meals.** These should never occur. The risks of hypoglycaemia are much reduced by ensuring that you have three proper meals, together with a mid-morning, mid-afternoon and bedtime snack. (On a four-a-day injection routine, the daytime snacks may not be needed but the bedtime snack is still essential.)

❖ **Accidental overdose of insulin.** If it does occur, this can usually be dealt with by taking extra carbohydrate. However, if you realise that an accidental overdose has been given which exceeds the usual dose by more than half, contact your doctor immediately for advice.

❖ **Increased physical activity.** This may not always be predictable, making it essential to have lump sugar, Dextrosol tablets or something similar at hand at all times (see question 15 on page 29).

❖ **Alcohol.** This can stop the body's automatic correction of hypoglycaemia. When drinking alcohol (especially spirits), ensure that you eat at the same time.

The body does have efficient built-in mechanisms for reversing mild to moderate hypoglycaemia but these should never be relied upon to correct this abnormal situation. Repeated attacks of severe hypoglycaemia can result in brain damage. Therefore, if you have frequent hypoglycaemia, mention it to your doctor so that you can be advised on the best course of action. **Hypoglycaemia is a preventable problem.**

25

How should hypoglycaemia be treated?

Firstly, as mentioned above, avoid hypo-glycaemia whenever possible. Always have a packet of Dextrosol in your pocket or handbag to correct minor hypoglycaemia, should it occur. More severe hypoglycaemia should be promptly corrected by an immediate snack of sweetened milk and a biscuit. Should you become drowsy and not able to take action yourself, your identification bracelet or pendant should enable others to provide force-feeding with a sweetened drink. **Hypostop** is a useful glucose-rich jelly which can be squeezed into your mouth or on your gums to correct hypoglycaemia. Failing this, a doctor will need to give you a glucose injection directly into a vein, and if no doctor is immediately on hand, no time should be wasted in having you transferred to the casualty department of the nearest hospital.

It is therefore essential that your family, friends, employers or other working colleagues should be made aware of the action they should take under such circumstances.

Glucagon, a hormone which has the opposite effect to insulin, is also available. If you tend to get severe episodes of hypoglycaemia, particularly if you live or are travelling somewhere remote from medical care, your doctor can supply ampoules of glucagon in a kit to be given to you in an emergency by a relative or friend. The usual dose is 1mg (in 1ml of solution) given by syringe into the muscle of the upper arm, just below the shoulder. A feeling of sickness occurs in some people given glucagon.

26

What are ketones and how does one test for them?

Body fat is both an insulator and a reserve store of energy. Whether you are diabetic or not, if you eat nothing for 12–18 hours, fat is broken down to provide this reserve energy. Some of the breakdown products of fat are substances called ketones, and these will appear in the urine under such circumstances. In the diabetic, however, ketones will also appear in the urine if diabetes goes badly out of control. This occurs because there is not enough insulin to provide the body cells with the energy (glucose) that they need: here again, the reserve energy (fat) stores are being called upon.

Ketones in the urine are a serious warning!

Ketones are most easily tested by Ketostix strips. Do the test whenever you feel ill in any way. If the result is positive, do the test again in four hours. If still positive, see your doctor immediately or contact your hotline number (see page 58).

What are ketoacidosis and diabetic coma?

If diabetic control remains poor, ketones cannot be excreted rapidly enough in the urine, and ketone levels will rise in the blood as well. Because ketones are acids, this affects the entire bodily function. Tiredness, drowsiness, sickness and vomiting can occur. In addition, by this time the large amount of glucose in the urine will cause an excessive loss of water. The mouth becomes dry, and breathing becomes deep and laboured. If no action is taken, coma develops. This whole sequence rarely occurs in less than 24 hours, so there is time to take avoiding action. Before the days of insulin, ketoacidosis was the major cause of death in people with diabetes. Today, provided ketoacidosis is identified and treated early, recovery is the rule. However, ketoacidosis is preventable.

Take action! If you are thirsty or passing more urine than usual, or if your blood glucose is over 17mmol/l at any time, you should immediately check for ketones. If the result is positive, test the urine again in four hours. If ketones are still present, contact your clinic, hospital or doctor, unless you have been given other specific instructions on dealing with this situation (see question 28 below).

How can ketoacidosis be prevented?

There is always a good reason for the loss of control which leads to ketoacidosis. The most common are: too much food or too little exercise; a forgotten or incorrect dose of insulin; other medication; infection and stress.

❖ **Food and exercise problems** are easily prevented by either avoiding changes in eating and exercise patterns, or increasing the dose of insulin when you increase food or reduce exercise. The amount by which you should increase the insulin is a matter of trial and error.

❖ **Your insulin requirements** can change over a period of time. Showing consistently higher blood glucose levels should prompt you to increase the dose of insulin by two to eight units, or contact your doctor or diabetes nurse.

❖ **A forgotten insulin dose** is not a disaster. If you are taking twice-daily insulin and you remember before your midday meal, give half to two-thirds of your usual dose then. If you only remember before your evening meal, check your urine or blood sugar and take advice, from either your doctor or your hotline, on what dose you should give . If on four injections a day and you miss one of your doses, it will produce a rise of blood glucose which is unlikely to cause you a problem; it is not usually worth adjusting the other doses.

❖ **Additional prescribed drugs** should always be discussed with your doctor to ensure that they do not interfere with diabetic control.

❖ **Infection and stress** are unavoidable aspects of life. Any stress, whether physical (an accident), mental (worry or depression) or medical (operations, infections or even a common cold), will cause some rise in blood glucose level to an extent which differs from person to person. Check your blood glucose every four to six hours while you are unwell. In any of these situations, the insulin may need to be increased by anything from two units to double the usual dose as soon as (or preferably before) blood glucose checks indicate a loss of control. You will get to know your own responses to these stresses, and discussion with your doctor will help to provide additional guidelines.

If your illness makes you vomit, feel sick, or you cannot eat, do not stop your insulin, but keep giving the same dose. Make sure that you test your blood glucose more frequently, since higher levels may prompt you to increase your insulin doses. Try to keep taking fluids which also provide some carbohydrate. The following foods may be useful if you are unwell because they provide concentrated carbohydrate in a liquid form to balance the effect of the insulin you are taking.

- ❖ sugar
- ❖ glucose
- ❖ jam/honey/marmalade
- ❖ Ribena (undiluted)
- ❖ orange squash (undiluted)
- ❖ orange juice
- ❖ lemonade
- ❖ Bournvita/Ovaltine
- ❖ milk pudding (tinned)
- ❖ drinking chocolate
- ❖ Complan (powder)
- ❖ Build-up (powder)

If ketones appear, contact the hotline number immediately (see page 58). If you remain ill for as long as six hours, arrange for someone to take you to the nearest hospital accident and emergency (casualty) department at once.

If your diabetes is seriously out of control and you are out of reach of all medical care, you may need to use an emergency measure to keep yourself out of trouble until medical advice is available. Give yourself 4 units of a fast-acting insulin such as Actrapid, Humulin-S or lispro every hour, also checking your blood sugar hourly until your glucose level returns to normal. It is also important to keep your fluid intake high – about 300–600ml (½–1 pint) of water per hour in the early stages.

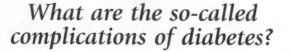

What are the so-called complications of diabetes?

Arteriosclerosis

Arteriosclerosis (hardening of the arteries) occurs to some extent in almost every person as they age, whether or not they are diabetic. In people with diabetes, it tends to occur somewhat earlier than usual. Arteriosclerosis is the cause of strokes and heart attacks. It may also produce poor circulation in the legs, which leads to painful calves on walking, poor healing of abrasions and blisters and occasionally gangrene. Hardening of the arteries is caused by fat being deposited in the walls of the arteries so that they become narrowed and even blocked. From time to time, your doctor will check the level of cholesterol (as well as other fats) in your blood. Keeping these blood fat levels normal is now known to reduce the risk of developing heart attacks and strokes. The way to keep the fat levels normal is to keep to the recommended diet (see question 8 on pages 14–18). Somewhat stricter dieting and even medicines may be prescribed for you if the fats in the blood test are found to be above safe levels. **People with diabetes should not smoke.** Smoking is the other big cause of hardening of the arteries. If arteries do become blocked, they can quite often be treated by a surgeon stretching or bypassing the block. But prevention is better than cure!

Cataracts

Cataracts are degenerative changes in the lens of the eye which can cause dimness of vision. Cataracts occur commonly in people without diabetes and somewhat more frequently in people with diabetes, especially if blood sugar levels are allowed to run high. Cataracts can be treated by quite a simple operation: the surgeon will usually replace your damaged lens with an artificial one.

Retinopathy

Retinopathy is the name given to leaky, and abnormally fragile, small blood vessels in the retina, the seeing part of the eye. In some people with diabetes such abnormalities may cause blurring, and occasionally loss of vision. In the early stages, however, you may not be aware that the retina is being damaged. It is therefore up to you to make sure that a doctor (or suitably qualified optician) checks your eyes every year with an ophthalmoscope. Drops will often be put in the eyes to widen the pupils and provide a better view of your retinas. Even once retinopathy has developed, it can be treated by using laser beam therapy – unless it is left too late. Again, think of prevention. Lower blood or urine glucose levels and a lower blood pressure mean a much lower risk of retinal damage.

Neuropathy

Neuropathy signifies nerve damage, which can cause weakness, pins and needles or a loss of feeling in the feet or hands. Some people have leg pains or feel that they are walking on cotton wool. You may not be aware that you have a loss of feeling in the feet; only a regular check by your doctor will make it possible to pick this problem up in its earliest form. Occasionally, dizziness and other unusual symptoms may occur. Even impotence can develop, although this may be due to factors other than diabetes. If you have this problem, do discuss it with your doctor, since many possible treatments for this are now available.

Nephropathy

Nephropathy means kidney damage, and may occur after long-standing diabetes. It is for this reason that your doctor checks for protein in your urine when you go for an appointment. If small quantities of a particular protein, albumin, are found in the urine, it is referred to as microalbuminuria. Your doctor may then recommend a drug known to reduce the risks of further kidney damage. A few people with advanced kidney damage may need dialysis (artificial kidney) treatment, or even a kidney transplant. Once again, think of prevention. The lower the blood (or urine) glucose and the lower the blood pressure, the better the chances of avoiding this problem.

Infection

Infection, particularly of the skin and urinary system, is more likely to occur in people with diabetes than in people without diabetes. In addition, healing of even minor injuries is sometimes slower. These problems are more likely to occur if your diabetes is not well controlled. Once infection occurs, it is essential that your diabetes control is improved to assist in the healing process

Foot ulcers

Foot ulcers are a particular risk. If feeling is lost, it is all too easy to be unaware of pressure on a toe or a minor injury. Repeated damage to this area, particularly if your blood circulation is poor, can then result in an ulcer. This can become more infected, producing swelling, redness and pain, and loss of control of your diabetes. You could become seriously ill, and gangrene may even develop, requiring amputation of part of your foot. Chronic ulcer infection can also damage the underlying bone, causing osteomyelitis. Once this sets in, long-term antibiotic treatment or surgery to your foot may prove necessary. Prevention is all-important; please read question 30 (below) very carefully. If you develop even the smallest weeping blister, ulcer or sore on your foot, let your doctor or diabetes nurse know immediately.

All the above complications can be effectively treated, particularly if detected early. It is for this reason that doctors will make a systematic examination of various parts of your body approximately once each year. You may need to remind them that this annual review is due.

How important is foot care?

The feet of a person with diabetes can be very vulnerable. Nerve damage (neuropathy) can prevent feeling an injury, scratch or cut; poor blood supply to the feet may then mean poor healing of the injury and infection, or gangrene can develop. The following rules are important to follow:

- ❖ Avoid walking barefoot, even at home.

- ❖ Do not cut your toenails too short, and cut nails to follow the line of the toe.

- ❖ Never cut your own toenails if you have a significant eyesight problem or a nerve or blood vessel disorder affecting the feet. See a state-registered chiropodist regularly, every six to eight weeks, if possible.

- ❖ Avoid tight shoes. Preferably have new shoes fitted by an expert who knows you are diabetic.

- ❖ Wash, dry and examine your feet carefully at least every other day. Even the most minor infection should be immediately discussed with your doctor.

- ❖ Never attempt to treat any foot problem yourself; permanent damage may result from the use of over-the-counter remedies. Always seek professional advice first.

RIGHT   **WRONG**

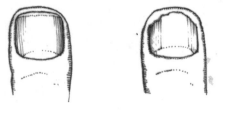

If an ulcer, sore or other foot infection develops, do not delay: contact your doctor immediately.

How will diabetes affect my lifestyle?

Can I smoke?
No! Diabetes alone may damage the blood vessels of your body, as mentioned earlier. If you smoke as well, your chances of such damage are that much greater.

Can I drive a car?
Yes, but the licensing authorities will need your doctor's reassurance that your diabetes is sufficiently stable and that you are otherwise well. You must let the DVLA know that you have diabetes.

Can I play sport as usual?
Yes (see questions 14 and 15 on pages 27–9).

Can I drink alcohol?
Yes, but as mentioned earlier, calories do count. In addition, if you are prone to having frequent hypos, alcohol (especially spirits) may block the body's corrective responses and make your hypos more severe. Remember that you should always have a carbohydrate snack if you have an alcoholic drink.

Does diabetes interfere with employment?
Hardly. Jobs involving physical responsibility for other people (such as bus and HGV drivers, airline pilots and certain branches of the armed forces), or involving personal danger

(working on high buildings, diving, and so on) are not suitable for insulin-receiving people with diabetes. Apart from these situations, there should be no problems. The earlier discrimination against people with diabetes is now almost non-existent since it has been shown that the work record of people with diabetes is no worse than the rest of the population.

Can I get life insurance?
Yes. You may have to accept a 'loading', but life assurance is possible for most people with diabetes. Shop around and seek advice from the British Diabetic Association.

Can I have children?

Yes. Diabetes is at least partly inherited. If either parent suffers from diabetes, the risk of any one child becoming diabetic at some time in their life is certainly greater than if this was not the case. However, the risk is not so high as to make having children unwise.

Pregnancy
Pregnancy in a diabetic person should always be managed by a physician-obstetrician team accustomed to dealing with diabetic pregnancies. If you are planning a family, let your doctor know. Together, you will be able to ensure that your control is as close as possible to perfection before you conceive. If you are practising contraception, your doctor will

advise you to continue this until your control is just right. You should wait until you get your doctor's go-ahead. This is now considered to be important in reducing many of the problems that may occur in diabetic pregnancy.

Contraception

Most of the presently available low-dose pills are satisfactory for people with diabetes and there is no reason why you cannot use a intra-uterine device (IUD) or other contraceptive methods. If you are taking the contraceptive pill, it is useful to stop it and to have one normal period before you conceive so that the exact duration of pregnancy is known. Your doctor and diabetes nurse will be happy to discuss any other aspects of diabetes and pregnancy with you.

33

When should I see my doctor or clinic nurse?

Ideally, you should have a discussion with them at least every three to four months. Do not forget to take your test record book with you when you go. At roughly annual intervals and perhaps more frequently, your doctor will systematically examine your eyes, blood pressure, heart and blood vessels on your feet, and check for nerve damage. Do not be afraid to remind them that your 12-monthly check is due. They will test the urine for protein and check the level of control of your diabetes and your kidney function and will probably take blood to see whether the blood fat (cholesterol and triglyceride) levels are normal. If they are not, an alteration to the diet, and perhaps tablets, may be suggested. As indicated earlier, a number of drugs in everyday use for other conditions may affect the control of your diabetes. Therefore, at these visits ask your doctor for reassurance that none of the other drugs that you are taking are interfering in any way. Each time you see either your family doctor or specialist, it is useful to take along your syringe or pen injector (it may need checking), your diet sheet (it may need changing) and your blood test record book (so that the doctor and nurse have information on the basis of which a change in treatment might be recommended).

In an emergency, if your tests show high sugar levels consistently, or if you begin to feel thirsty or unwell, do not wait – get advice. Make sure that you have one or more telephone numbers that you or your family or friends may contact for advice on such unexpected problems, and write them down in the space provided at the end of this book (see page 59).

Are any new treatments under development?

Insulin can now be implanted in refillable reservoirs beneath the skin and delivered into body tissues with a mini-pump regulated by a remote control. Priming of the reservoir through the skin is only required every week or so. Although this is not actually an artificial pancreas, such a concept is getting closer. Diabetic control achieved in this way is not necessarily better than with multiple injections. The pumps are very expensive and require special training both for the patient and the staff responsible for caring for you.

Pancreas transplantation is now being carried out more widely, usually only when a kidney is being transplanted. It has a better than 50 per cent success rate but has the drawback of needing immuno-suppression. This involves drugs that themselves bring problems.

Methods of giving insulin more comfortably, by inhalation, nasal spray or air-jet, are also under development.

What should I do about identification?

Always carry a card, or better still, a bracelet or pendant, indicating that you have diabetes. In this day and age, accidents will happen, and it is obviously important that anyone can immediately identify you as being diabetic. The Medicalert Foundation (local address available from your doctor), which provides identification bracelets and pendants at a modest cost, now has branches in many countries. This system is highly recommended. Alternatively, have your local jeweller make one for you.

Where can I get support?

A lot of people with diabetes feel over-whelmed by what they need to know and do. It is quite common to feel low or anxious from time to time, both about the present and the future. Make a point of building up links with a diabetes nurse or your doctor so that you know whom to consult if the going gets a bit rough. Your doctor, dietitian, diabetes nurse or chiropodist/podiatrist will be only too happy to clear up any uncertainties.

Being a member of the British Diabetic Association (see page 59) has much to offer. It provides a care and helpline too Its monthly magazine, *Balance*, will help you follow recent trends in diabetes care. A lot of research is also being carried out in diabetes. You will find it useful and interesting to keep in touch with these and other important developments. If you are a youngster or teenager, the association provides group activities in which you may enjoy participating.

Hotline number

Keep a record here of a telephone number from which you can get advice 24 hours a day, seven days a week, should any sudden problem occur that affects your diabetes. Your doctor will advise you which number to insert.

Other important contact numbers

Your family doctor . . . .

Your hospital clinic . . . .

Your dietitian . . . .

Your chiropodist/podiatrist . . . .

Your diabetic advisory nurse . . . .

The British Diabetic Association 0171 323 1531

Some books for further reading and reference

Living with Diabetes – Type 1 Diabetes by
Dr J. Day (John Wiley and Sons)

Diabetes at Your Fingertips by P. Sonksen,
C. Fox and S. Judd (Class Publishing)

Creative Recipes for All Occasions (BDA
Publications)

So Your Child Has Diabetes by B. Estridge and
J. Davies

Index